I want to thank you and congratulate you for downloading the book,

"Pharmacology Nursing Review".

By

Anna Curran. RN-BC, BSN, PHN, CMSRN

Emergency Room Registered Nurse

Critical Care Transport Nurse

Clinical Nurse Instructor for LVN and BSN students

Anna began writing materials to help her BSN and LVN students with their studies. She takes the topics that the students are learning and expands on them to try to help with their understanding of the nursing process. Her experience spans over 2 decades in nursing, starting as an LVN in 1993. She received her RN license in 1997. She has worked in Medical-Surgical, Telemetry, ICU and the ER. She found a passion in the ER and has stayed in this department for 16 years. She is a clinical instructor for LVN and BSN students along with a critical care transport nurse.

Practice tests and review make all the difference in the world when testing. This book is to supplement your other study materials. Review of Pharmacology will increase your retention.

Free bonus test in this book 74 Medical Surgical questions with rationale to the link below

http://nursestudy.net/practice-exams-list/

Visit us at: **http://nursestudy.net/**

Thanks again for purchasing this book. If you like the book please leave us feedback and let us know.

Table of Contents

Visit us at NurseStudy.Net

Angiotensin Converting Enzyme (ACE) Inhibitors

Description

Slows the activity of the angiotensin converting enzyme (ACE), lowers the production of angiotensin II, causing blood vessels to relax and dilate, blood pressure lowers, and more oxygen-rich blood reaches the heart.

Used to treat:

Hypertension, MI, Stroke

Examples: Usually end in "Pril"

benazepril (Lotensin)

captopril (Capoten)

enalapril (Vasotec)

fosinopril (Monopril)

lisinopril (Prinivil, Zestril)

moexipril (Univasc)

perindopril (Aceon)

quinapril (Accupril)

ramipril (Altace)

trandolapril (Mavik)

Quick Med Fact:

This medication can cause a dry cough.

Angiotensin Receptor Blockers (ARBs)

Description

These medications block the action of angiotensin II by preventing angiotensin II from binding to angiotensin II receptors on blood vessels. As a result, blood vessels dilate and blood pressure drops.

Used to treat:

Hypertension and CHF

Slow the progression of kidney disease due to high blood pressure or diabetes.

Examples: Usually end in "Sartan"

candesartan (Atacand)

irbesartan (Avapro)

losartan (Cozaar)

olmesartan* (Benicar)

valsartan* (Diovan)

Quick Med Fact:

Sometimes used for patients who are not able to take Ace Inhibitors

Anti-Alzheimer's Agents

DESCRIPTION

These medications:

May prevent the breakdown of acetylcholine by blocking the activity of acetylcholinesterase (cholinesterase inhibitors).

Help regulate the activity of glutamate, a chemical involved in the processing, storage and retrieval of information (NMDA receptor antagonists).

Used to treat:

Used to manage Alzheimer's

EXAMPLES

cholinesterase inhibitor

donepezil* (Aricept)

galantamine (Razadyne)

rivastigmine (Exelon)

NMDA receptor antagonist

memantine* (Namenda)

Quick Med Fact:

These medications will only slow down the symptoms getting worse. There is no cure for Alzheimer's.

Anti-Infectives – Aminoglycosides

DESCRIPTION

Bactericidal; work by blocking protein synthesis in bacteria and breakdown the structure of the bacterial cell wall.

Used to treat:

Severe infections, (i.e UTI, and Septicemia).

Klebsiella species

 Escherichia coli Klebsiella species.

EXAMPLES

amikacin (Amikin)

gentamicin (Garamycin)

kanamycin (Kantrex)

neomycin (Neo-Fradin)

streptomycin (Streptomycin)

tobramycin (Nebcin, TOBI)

Quick Med Fact:

Can be very Ototoxic and Nephrotoxic

Anti-Infectives – Cephalosporins

DESCRIPTION

These antibiotics are broad spectrum made from the mold Cephalosporium. Like penicillins, they interfere with bacterial cell wall synthesis.

Used to treat:

A variety of bacterial infections, including respiratory tract infections, skin, & urinary tract infections.

EXAMPLES

1st Generation

cefadroxil (Duricef)

ceFAZolin (Ancef)

cephalexin* (Keflex)

2nd Generation

cefaclor (Raniclor, Ceclor)

cefOXitin (Mefoxin)

cefprozil (Cefzil)

cefuroxime (Ceftin, Zinacef)

3rd Generation

cefdinir* (Omnicef)

cefixime (Suprax)

cefoperazone (Cefobid)

cefotaxime (Claforan)

cefpodoxime (Vantin)

cefTAZidime (Fortaz, Tazicef)

ceftibuten (Cedax)

ceftizoxime (Cefizox)

cefTRIAXone (Rocephin)

4th Generation

cefepime (Maxipime)

Quick Med Fact:

Have been used for patients with allergy to PCN. Can be 3 x more effective than PCN in treating infections of the throat, example: strep throat.

Anti-Infectives – Fluoroquinolones

DESCRIPTION

These medications are bactericidal; they are the only class of antimicrobial agents in clinical use that directly inhibit DNA synthesis in bacteria.

Used to treat:

Infections such as sinuses, skin, lungs, ears, airways, urinary tract, bones, and joints caused by gram negative and gram positive organisms.

Prevent and treat anthrax.

EXAMPLES

ciprofloxacin (Cipro)

gatifloxacin (Tequin)

levofloxacin* (Levaquin)

moxifloxacin* (Avelox)

norfloxacin (Noroxin)

Quick Med Fact:

Can also be used to fight again illnesses that are caused by biological warfare (Plague and Anthrax).

Did you know that these medications can increase the chances of tendonitis and tendon rupture in patients?

Anti-Infectives – Macrolides

DESCRIPTION

Bacteriostatic. Inhibits bacterial growth and reproduction by interfering with their ability to make proteins.

Used to treat:

Localized and systemic bacterial infections of the respiratory tract, gastrointestinal tract, and soft tissues.

Treat severe acne and sexually transmitted infections.

Prevent whopping cough, as well as endocarditis in dentistry.

EXAMPLES

azithromycin (Zithromax)

clarithromycin (Biaxin)

dirithromycin (Dynabac)

erythromycin (E-Mycin)

troleandomycin (Tao)

Quick Med Fact:

Can be used in patients with PCN allergies.

Elderly patients who take calcium channel blockers can become hypotensive or shock if they take erythromycin or clarithromycin. If macrolide is needed, azithromycin may be an option.

Anti-Infectives – Penicillins

DESCRIPTION

These medications belong to a class of antibiotics called beta-lactams, which exert bactericidal action by inhibiting bacterial cell wall production. Currently this group includes more than 20 antibiotics.

Used to treat:

A wide range of bacterial infections including streptococcal infections, syphilis and Lyme disease.

EXAMPLES

Amoxicillin (Amoxil)

ampicillin (Principen, Omnipen)

Extended spectrum penicillins

carbenicillin (Geocillin)

piperacillin (Pipracil)

ticarcillin (Ticar)

Natural penicillins

penicillin G (generic)

penicillin V (Pen-VK)

Penicillinase-resistant penicillins

dicloxacillin (Dynapen)

nafcillin (generic)

oxacillin (generic)

Quick Med Fact:

Potassium sparing diuretics and ACE inhibitors can increase the risk of hyperkalemia when given with PCN.

Anti-Infectives – Sulfonamides

DESCRIPTION

These bacteriostatic medications provide a broad spectrum of activity against both gram-positive and gram-negative bacteria.

Used to treat:

Treat urinary tract infections.

Treat some types of bacterial pneumonia (*Pneumocystis Carinii*) and shigellosis.

Treat some protozoal infections.

EXAMPLES

mafenide (Sulfamylon)

sulfacetamide ophthalmic (Bleph 10)

sulfamethizole (Thiosulfil Forte)

sulfaSALAzine (Azulfidine)

sulfisoxazole (Gantrisin)

trimethoprim-sulfamethoxazole* (Septra, Bactrim)

Quick Med Fact:

Avoid taking with herbs with diuretic effect

Anti-Infectives – Tetracyclines

DESCRIPTION

Broad spectrum anti-infectives, their bacteriostatic effect by inhibiting protein synthesis in bacteria.

Used to treat:

Respiratory tract infections.

Treat acne and skin infections, genital infections (syphilis, chlamydia), and urinary tract infections.

Treat Lyme disease, mycoplasmal infections and rickettsial infections and the infection that causes stomach ulcers (caused by *Helicobacter pylori*).

EXAMPLES

demeclocycline (Declomycin)

doxycycline* (Vibramycin)

minocycline (Minocin)

oxytetracycline (Terramycin)

tetracycline (Sumycin)

Quick Med Fact:

Take on empty stomach.

Do not give to pregnant women or children under 8 years old as they can stain developing teeth, including in fetus.

Do not take with milk.

Antianginals – Nitrates

DESCRIPTION

Vasodilators dilate the blood vessels, improve blood flow and allow more oxygen-rich blood to reach the heart muscle. They also relax the veins.

Used to treat:

Angina.

EXAMPLES

isosorbide dinitrate (Dilatrate-SR, Sorbitrate, Isordil)

isosorbide mononitrate* (ISMO, Monoket, Imdur)

nitroglycerin (Nitro-Dur, Nitro-Bid, Nitrostat)

Quick Med Fact:

Patients should not take Viagra, Levitra, or Cialis within 24-36 hours of taking Nitrates.

Can cause headaches, hypotension, and dizziness.

Antianxiety Agents

DESCRIPTION

These medications act at many levels in the central nervous system (CNS), producing an anxiolytic effect. They may produce CNS depression. The effects may be mediated by GABA (an inhibitory neurotransmitter).

Used to treat:

Generalized Anxiety Disorder (GAD) & Panic Disorders.

Manage anxiety associated with depression.

EXAMPLES

Antidepressants (SSRI)

PARoxetine* (Paxil)

venlafaxine* (Effexor)

Antidepressants (tricyclic)

doxepin (SINEquan)

Antihistamine

hydrOXYzine (Atarax, Vistaril)

Benzodiazepines

ALPRAZolam* (Xanax)

busPIRone (Buspar, Vanspar)

chlordiazePOXIDE (Librium)

diazepam* (Valium)

LORazepam* (Ativan)

! midazolam (Versed)

oxazepam (Serax)

Herbals

kava-kava (herbal)

lemon verbena (herbal)

valerian (herbal)

Tranquilizer

meprobomate (Equanil)

Quick Med Fact:

Valerian is used as a sleep aid. It should be stopped 1 week prior to surgery as it may interact with anesthesia.

Antiarrhythmics

DESCRIPTION

Generally classified by their effects on cardiac conduction tissue (Class IA, IB, IC, II, III, IV). They:

Slow down the heart (the calcium channel blockers, digoxin, and beta-blockers).

Slow the heart's electrical impulses by blocking the heart's potassium channels (amiodarone, sotalol, dofetilide).

Used to treat:

Suppress potentially lethal cardiac arrhythmias.

EXAMPLES

Class IA

disopyramide (Norpace)

procainamide (Pronestyl)

quiNIDine (Quinidine Sulfate)

Class IB

 lidocaine (Xylocaine)

mexiletine (Mexitil)

phenytoin (Dilantin)

Class IC

flecainide (Tambocor)

propafenone (Rythmol)

Class II (Beta-blockers)

acebutolol (Sectral)

 propranolol (Inderal)

sotalol (Betapace)

Class III

amiodarone (Cordarone)

dofetilide (Tikosyn)

ibutilide (Convert)

Class IV (Calcium-channel blockers)

diltiazem* (Cardizem, Dilacor, Tiazac, and others)

verapamil* (Calan, Covera, Isoptin, Verelan)

Other

digoxin* (Lanoxin)

dronedarone (Multaq)

Quick Med Fact:

Amiodarone can cause skin to take on a blue/gray color. This can go away when medication has been stopped and some time has passed.

Patients with low potassium levels can develop digoxin toxicity.

Antiasthmatics

DESCRIPTION

These medications:

Relax the smooth muscles that line the airway (bronchodilators).

Block the inflammation that narrows the airways (corticosteroids).

Counteract substances that cause the air passages to constrict and secrete mucus (leukotriene modifiers).

Prevent allergic reactions or asthma symptoms.

Uses to treat:

Manage acute and chronic episodes of reversible bronchoconstriction associated with asthma.

Treat acute attacks (short-term control) and decrease incidence and intensity of future attacks (long-term control).

EXAMPLES

Adrenergics

albuterol* (Proventil, Ventolin, Proair, AccuNeb)

EPINEPHrine (EpiPen, Primatene, Nephron, Adrenalin)

Bronchodilators

theophylline (Theo-Dur, Slo-Bid, Aerolate, and others)

Corticosteriods

budesonide (Entocort EC, Pulmicort)

ciclesonide (Omnaris)

Herbals

eucalyptus (herbal)

Leukotriene antagonists

montelukast (Singulair)

zafirlukast (Accolate)

Mast cell stabilizers

cromolyn nebulized solution (NasalCrom)

Monoclonal antibodies

omalizumab (Xolair)

Other

albuterol & ipratropium (Combivent)

Quick Med Fact:

Patients should use Albuterol first.

Epipen can be injected directly through clothing, outer thigh, hold in place for 10 minutes to make sure all medication is delivered.

Anticoagulants

DESCRIPTION

Inhibits clotting factor synthesis, inhibits thrombin, and/or interferes with blood platelet formation.

Used to treat:

Treatment and prevention of blood clots associated with stroke, heart attack, heart valve disease, coronary artery disease, heart failure, arrhythmia, atrial fibrillation, deep vein thrombosis, and pulmonary embolism.

EXAMPLES

heparin (generic)

warfarin (Coumadin)

LMWH

dalteparin (Fragmin)

enoxaparin (Lovenox)

tinzaparin (Innohep)

Thrombin inhibitors

argatroban (generic)

bivalirudin (Angiomax)

dabigatran (Pradaxa)

desirudin (Iprivask)

lepirudin (rDNA)

Quick Med Fact:

Green and leafy foods are rich in vitamin K and can reduce the effectiveness of anticoagulant therapy.

Certain herbal remedies and increase and decrease the PT/INR levels.

Anticonvulsants

DESCRIPTION

These medications depress central nervous system function. They target specific neurochemical processes, suppress excess neuron function, and regulate electrochemical signals in the brain (for instance, GABA inhibitors).

Used to treat:

Help control epileptic seizures.

Treats neuropathic pain (associated with diabetes, shingles, and fibromyalgia), migraine headaches, and bipolar disorder.

EXAMPLES

Barbiturates

mephobarbital (Mebaral)

PENTobarbital (Nembutal)

PHENobarbital (Luminal, Solfoton)

Benzodiazepines

clonazePAM (KlonoPIN)

clorazepate (Tranxene)

diazepam (Valium)

GABA analogues

gabapentin (Neurontin)

pregabalin (Lyrica)

tiaGABine (Gabitril)

Hydantoins

ethotoin (Peganone)

fosphenytoin (Cerebyx)

phenytoin (Dilantin)

Other

carBAMazepine (TEGretol)

lamoTRIgine (LaMICtal)

OXcarbazepine (Trileptal)

topiramate (Topamax)

valproic acid (Depakote)

Oxazolidinediones

trimethadione (Tridione)

Quick Med Fact:

Some anticonvulsants can cause SJS or toxic epidural syndrome. Notify MD immediately at first sign of rash.

May increase sensitivity to sunlight.

Antidepressants – Monoamine Oxidase Inhibitors (MAOIs)

DESCRIPTION

Prevents the enzyme monamine oxidase from breaking down the neurotransmitters norepinephrine and serotonin (also known as monoamines) in the brain.

Used to treat:

Treat depression.

EXAMPLES

isocarboxazid (Marplan)

phenelzine (Nardil)

selegiline (Ensam, Eldepryl, Zelapar)

tranylcypromine (Parnate)

Quick Med Fact:

DO not mix with tyramine as it can sharply increase blood pressure.

Taking St. John's wort can raise serotonin levels to dangerously high levels (serotonin syndrome).

Antidepressants – Selective Serotonin Reuptake Inhibitors (SSRIs)

DESCRIPTION

These medications block the reabsorption (reuptake) of serotonin.

Used to treat:

Used to treat moderate-to-severe depression and chronic fatigue syndrome.

Treat premenstrual dysphoric disorder, obsessive-compulsive disorder, panic disorder, post-traumatic stress disorder, and generalized anxiety disorder.

EXAMPLES

citalopram (CeleXA)

escitalopram (Lexapro)

FLUoxetine (PROzac)

PARoxetine (Paxil)

sertraline (Zoloft)

Quick Med Fact:

Weight gain of 10 + pounds is not uncommon with this medication.

All antidepressants can cause increased risk of suicidal thinking.

Antidepressants – Serotonin and Norepinephrine Reuptake Inhibitors (SNRIs)

DESCRIPTION

Block or delay the reuptake of serotonin and norepinephrine by the presynaptic nerves. The increased levels of these neurotransmitters elevates mood.

Used to treat:

Depression, anxiety disorder, panic disorder and other mood disorders.

EXAMPLES

desvenlafaxine (Pristiq)

duloxetine (Cymbalta)

milnacipran (Savella)

venlafaxine (Effexor)

Quick Med Fact:

Increased risk of bleeding if taken with aspirin, NSAIDS, and/or anticoagulants.

Antidepressants – Tricyclic & Tetracyclic

DESCRIPTION

Inhibits the nerve cell's ability to reuptake serotonin and norepinephrine, causing increased levels of these neurotransmitters in the brain. They also block the action of acetylcholine and histamine (causing many of the side effects of these meds).

Used to treat:

Depression and help treat OCD and bedwetting.

Off-label uses include panic disorder, bulimia, and chronic pain (migraine, diabetic neuropathy & post-herpetic neuralgia).

EXAMPLES

amitriptyline (Elavil)

amoxapine (Asendin)

desipramine (Norpramin)

doxepin (SINEquan)

imipramine (Tofranil)

maprotiline (Ludiomil)

nortriptyline (Pamelor)

protriptyline (Vivactil)

trimipramine (Surmontil)

Quick Med Fact:

Can cause restlessness and anxiousness.

One of the leading causes of death by overdose.

Antidiabetics – Insulins

DESCRIPTION

Used in the treatment of type 1 diabetes mellitus and may be used to treat type 2 diabetes mellitus.

Uses:

Rapid-acting insulin covers meals eaten at the same time as the injection.

Short-acting insulin covers meals eaten within 30 to 60 minutes.

Intermediate-acting insulin covers about half of the day or overnight (and is often combined with rapid- or short-acting insulin).

Long-acting insulin covers about one full day.

EXAMPLES

Intermediate-acting

NPH insulin (N) (HumuLIN-N, NovoLIN-N)

Long-acting

insulin detemir (Levemir)

insulin glargine (Lantus)

Rapid-acting

insulin aspart (NovoLOG)

insulin glulisine (Apidra)

insulin lispro (HumaLOG)

Short-acting

human insulin (Velosulin)

regular insulin (R) (HumuLIN-R, NovoLIN)

Quick Med Fact:

Regular insulin is the only insulin is the only one that can be given IV. The nurse will need to monitor blood glucose very carefully.

Antidiabetics – Oral Agents

DESCRIPTION

Stimulate insulin release from the beta cells of the pancreas (sulfonylureas and meglitinides).

Improve insulin's ability to move glucose into cells, especially muscle cells (biguanides).

Enhance insulin effectiveness in both muscle and adipose tissue (thiazolidinediones).

Block enzymes that help digest starches, slowing the rise in blood sugar (alpha-glucosidase inhibitors)

Block an enzyme that deactivates a protein (GLP-1), which will keep insulin circulating in the blood (DPP-4 inhibitors).

Used to treat:

Treat type 2 diabetes mellitus.

EXAMPLES

Alpha-Glucosidase Inhibitors

acarbose (Precose)

miglitol (Glyset)

Biguanides

metFORMIN (Glucophage)

Dipeptidyl peptidase-4 (DPP-4) inhibitors

sitaGLIPtin (Januvia)

Meglitinides

nateglinide (Starlix)

repaglinide (Prandin)

Sulfonylureas

glimepiride (Amaryl)

glipiZIDE (Glucotrol)

glyBURIDE (DiaBeta, Micronase)

Thiazolidinediones

pioglitazone (Actos)

rosiglitazone (Avandia)

Quick Med Fact:

Glyburide can cause sunburn more easily. Advice patients to wear sunblock of SPH 30 or higher.

Antidiarrheals

DESCRIPTION

Slows the passage of stools through the intestines (loperamide).

Decreases the secretion of fluid into the intestine and inhibit the activity of bacteria (bismuth subsalicylate).

Used to treat:

Control acute and chronic nonspecific diarrhea.

EXAMPLES

bismuth subsalicylate (Kaopectate, Pepto-Bismol)

diphenoxylate & atropine (Lomotil)

kaolin & pectin (Kapectolin)

Antispasmodics

loperamide (Imodium A-D)

Bulk-forming laxatives

polycarbophil (Equalactin, FiberCon)

Opiate

paregoric (generic)

Somatostatin analog

octreotide (SandoSTATIN)

Quick Med Fact:

Bismuth can cause dark tint in stool and tongue.

Do not give to children can cause Reye's syndrome

Antiemetics

DESCRIPTION

Inhibit the chemoreceptor trigger zone in the medulla by blocking dopamine receptors.

Decrease the sensitivity of the vestibular apparatus (for example, meclizine).

Block the effects of serotonin in the brain and small intestine.

Used to treat:

Various causes of nausea and vomiting, including surgery, anesthesia, antineoplastic and radiation therapies, and motion sickness.

EXAMPLES

5-HT3 antagonists

dolasetron (Anzemet)

granisetron (Sancuso)

nabilone (Cesamet)

ondansetron (Zofran)

palonosetron (Aloxi)

Anticholinergics

scopolamine (Transderm-Scop)

Cannabinoids

dronabinol (Marinol)

Herbals

ginger (herbal)

Neurokinin antagonists

aprepitant (Emend)

Other

dimenhyDRINATE (Dramamine, Dimetabs)

meclizine (Antivert, Bonine)

metoclopramide (Reglan)

Phenothiazines

chlorproMAZINE (Thorazine)

perphenazine (Trilafon)

prochlorperazine (Compro)

promethazine (Phenergan)

thiethylperazine (Norzine, Torecan)

Quick Med Fact:

Chlorpromazine can be used to treat intractable hiccups.

Antifungals

Also known as antimycotic agents. They destroy or inactivate fungi.

Used to treat:

Treat systemic, localized, or topical fungal infections (including yeast infections).

EXAMPLES

Azole antifungals (the triazoles and imidazoles)

butoconazole (Gynazole)

clotrimazole (Lotrisone)

fluconazole* (Diflucan)

itraconazole (Sporanox)

ketoconazole (Feoris, Nizoral)

miconazole (Aloe Vesta, Cruex)

oxiconazole (Oxistat)

posaconazole (Noxafil)

sertaconazole (Ertaczo)

sulconazole (Exelderm)

tioconazole (Monistat-1)

voriconazole (Vfend)

Echinocandins

anidulafungin (Eraxis)

caspofungin (Cancidas)

micafungin (Mycamine)

Herbals

goldenseal (herbal)

Miscellaneous antifungals

butenafine (Mentax)

ciclopirox (Loprox, Penlac Nail Lacquer)

flucytosine (Ancobon)

terbinafine (LamISIL)

tolnaftate (Absorbine Jr.)

Polyenes

amphotericin B deoxycholate (Amphocin, Fungizone)

nystatin (Mycostatin)

Quick Med Fact:

Fungi can survive for long periods, because of this fact, patients may need to take medications for a long period of time.

Can cause liver damage.

Antihistamines

DESCRIPTION

Competes with histamine for histamine receptor sites. By occupying the histamine receptor sites, they prevent histamine from causing allergic symptoms.

Used to treat:

Relief of symptoms associated with allergies (including rhinitis, urticaria and angioedema).

Adjunctive therapy in anaphylactic reactions.

Treat insomnia (diphenhydramine), motion sickness (dimenhydrinate and meclizine), Parkinson-like reactions (diphenhydramine), and other nonallergic conditions.

EXAMPLES

azelastine (Astelin)

bepotastine (Bepreve)

cetirizine (Zyrtec)

chlorpheniramine (Chlor-Trimeton)

clemastine (Tavist Allergy)

cyproheptadine (Periactin)

desloratadine (Clarinex)

dimenhyDRINATE (Dramamine, Dimetabs)

diphenhydrAMINE (Benadryl, Sominex, Nytol, Midol PM, Unisom Nighttime Sleep-Aid)

doxepin (SINEquan)

fexofenadine (Allegra)

hydrOXYzine (Atarax, Vistaril)

levocetirizine (Xyzal)

loratadine (Alavert, Claritin, Tavist ND, Dimetapp ND)

meclizine (Antivert, Bonine, Dramamine Less Drowsy Formula)

olopatadine nasal spray (Patanase)

! promethazine (Phenergan)

triprolidine (Zymine)

Quick Med Fact:

Antihistamines appear on the Beers List (medications inappropriate for the elderly)

Elderly at risk for orthostatic hypotension.

Antihyperuricemics

DESCRIPTION

Also called antigout agents, these medications work to either correct overproduction or underexcretion of uric acid.

Used to treat:

Gout

EXAMPLES

allopurinol (Zyloprim)

pegloticase (Krystexxa)

rasburicase (Elitek)

Quick Med Fact:

Patient may have an increased amount of gout flare ups when they first start these meds.

Antineoplastics

DESCRIPTION

Inhibits and/ or prevents development, maturation or spread of neoplastic cells by various different mechanisms of action.

Damage the DNA of cancer cells.

Interfere with the cancer cell's metabolism or affect cell division.

Create an unfavorable environment for cancer cell growth (hormones).

Used to treat:

Various solid tumors, lymphomas, and leukemias.

Prescribed for some autoimmune disorders (such as rheumatoid arthritis).

EXAMPLES

Alkylating agents

chlorambucil (Leukeran)

cyclophosphamide (Cytoxan, Endoxan, Neosar)

Antiestrogens

tamoxifen (Soltamox)

Antimetabolites

5-fluorouracil (5-FU)

methotrexate (Rheumatrex, Trexall)

Antitumor antibiotics

mitomycin (generic)

Enzymes

asparaginase (Elspar)

Human recombinant interleukin-2

aldesleukin (Proleukin)

Monoclonal antibodies

alemtuzumab (Campath)

trastuzumab (Herceptin)

Plant alkaloids

vinBLAStine (Velban)

vinCRIStine (Oncovin)

Quick Med Fact:

Healthcare workers should limit exposure to these medications. Healthcare workers need proper training before handling these medications.

Antiparkinson Agents

DESCRIPTION

These medications replenish dopamine. They also mimic the role of dopamine or block the effects of other chemicals that cause problems in the brain when dopamine levels drop.

Used to treat:

Relieve the symptoms of parkinsonism including tremor or trembling in the hands, arms, legs, jaw, and face; stiffness or rigidity of the arms, legs, and trunk; bradykinesia; poor balance and coordination.

EXAMPLES

biperiden (Akineton)

Anticholinergics

benztropine (Cogentin)

trihexyphenidyl (Artane, Trihexane)

Carbidopa/levodopa therapy

carbidopa & levodopa (Sinemet)

COMT inhibitors

entacapone (Comtan)

tolcapone (Tasmar)

Dopamine agonists

apomorphine (Apokyn)

bromocriptine (Parlodel)

pramipexole (Mirapex)

rOPINIrole (Requip)

rotigotine (Neupro)

MAO-B inhibitors

rasagiline (Azilect)

selegiline (Ensam, Eldepryl, Zelapar)

Other

amantadine (Symmetrel)

rivastigmine (Exelon)

Quick Med Fact:

On-off phenomenon is when the helpful effects wear off, alternative treatments will need to be started.

Antiplatelet Agents

DESCRIPTION

Blocks the formation of blood clots by preventing the clumping of platelets.

Used to treat:

Prevents and treats thromboembolic events, such as stroke, myocardial infarction, or peripheral vascular disease.

Prescribed after devices are placed inside the heart or blood vessels, such stents and artificial heart values.

EXAMPLES

aspirin (Bayer)

cilotazol

Adenosine diphosphate (ADP) receptor inhibitors

clopidogrel (Plavix)

prasugrel (Effient)

ticlopidine (Ticlid)

Adenosine reuptake inhibitors

dipyridamole (Persantine)

Glycoprotein IIb IIIa inhibitors

abciximab (ReoPro)

eptifibatide (Integrilin)

tirofiban (Aggrastat)

Herbals

ginkgo (herbal)

Phosphodiesterase inhibitors

cilostazol (Pletal)

Quick Med Fact:

Clients with heart failure should not take Cilostazol.

Antipsychotics

DESCRIPTION

Blocks a specific subtype of the dopamine receptor (the D2 receptor). The 2nd generation not only block D2 receptors, but also a specific subtype of serotonin receptor (5HR2A receptor).

Used to treat:

Acute and chronic psychosis, especially when accompanied by increased psychomotor activity.

Off-label uses include Tourette's syndrome, substance abuse, stuttering, obsessive-compulsive disorder, post-traumatic stress disorder, depression, bipolar disorder and personality disorders.

EXAMPLES

Atypical (or 2nd generation) antipsychotics

aripiprazole (Abilify)

clozapine (Clozaril)

olanzapine (ZyPREXA)

paliperidone (Invega)

QUEtiapine (SEROquel)

risperiDONE (RisperDAL)

ziprasidone (Geodon)

Others

iloperidone (Fanapt)

prochlorperazine (Compro)

thioridazine (Mellaril)

Typical antipsychotics

chlorproMAZINE (Thorazine)

fluphenazine (Permitil, Prolixin)

haloperidol (Haldol)

loxapine (Loxitane)

molindone (Moban)

perphenazine (Trilafon)

pimozide (Orap)

thiothixene (Navane)

trifluoperazine (Stelazine)

Quick Med Fact:

Watch for extrapyramidal effects.

Possible metabolism changes and weight gain.

Antirheumatics

DESCRIPTION

Treat rheumatoid arthritis. They relieve pain (analgesics), reduce inflammation (NSAIDs & steroids), and control the underlying disease (disease modifying rheumatoid arthritis drugs or DMARDs & biologic drugs).

Used to treat:

rheumatoid arthritis (RA) by slowing down joint destruction and preserving joint function (DMARDs).

Target specific components of the immune system (biologic agents - IM or IV only). These may be used alone, but are often given with other DMARDs to increase the benefits and limit potential side effects.

EXAMPLES

Biologic response modifiers (anti-TNF)

adalimumab (Humira)

certolizumab pegol (Cimzia)

etanercept (Enbrel)

golimumab (Simponi)

inFLIXimab (Remicade)

DMARDs

azathioprine (Imuran, Azasan)

cycloSPORINE (Neoral, SandIMMUNE)

gold sodium thiomalate (Myochrysine)

hydroxychloroquine (Plaquenil)

leflunomide (Arava)

methotrexate (Rheumatrex, Trexall)

sulfaSALAzine (Azulfidine)

Other biologics

abatacept (Orencia)

anakinra (Kineret)

riTUXimab (Rituxan)

tocilizumab (Actemra)

Quick Med Fact:

Sulfasalazine may turn urine, tears and sweat orange.

Antituberculars

DESCRIPTION

Have various actions that affect mycobacteria, with most having bactericidal (for example, rifampin) and/or bacteriostatic (for example, isoniazid) actions.

Used to treat:

Treat and prevent tuberculosis (TB).

EXAMPLES

Combination drugs

rifampin & isoniazid & pyrazinamide (Rifater)

Primary agents

ethionamide (Trecator SC)

isoniazid (INH, Nydrazid)

rifampin (Rifadin)

rifapentine (Priftin)

Second line agents

capreomycin (Capastat)

cycloSERINE (Seromycin)

ethambutol (Myambutol)

pyrazinamide (PZA) (generic)

streptomycin (generic)

Third line agents (Aminoglycosides)

kanamycin (Kantrex)

Quick Med Fact:

Rifampin can cause reddish orange discoloration of feces, sweat, urine, saliva, and skin.

Antiulcer Agents

DESCRIPTION

Blocks secretion of gastric acid by the gastric parietal cells (PPIs). They also stop the action of histamine on the gastric parietal cells, which inhibits the secretion of gastric acid (H-2 receptor blockers).

Used to treat:

Prevention and treatment of peptic ulcer and gastric hypersecretory conditions, e.g., Zollinger-Ellison syndrome.

Manage the symptoms of gastroesophageal reflux disease (GERD).

Treat recurrent gastric and duodenal ulcers caused by *Helicobacter pylori* infections (a combined antibiotic and gastric acid suppression therapy).

EXAMPLES

Anti-infective (Penicillins)

amoxicillin (Amoxil)

Herbal

comfrey (herbal)

Histamine H2-receptor antagonists

cimetidine (Tagamet)

famotidine (Pepcid)

nizatidine (Axid)

ranitidine (Zantac)

Mucosal protective

aluminum hydroxide (Amphojel)

aluminum hydroxide & magnesium hydroxide (Maalox, Mylanta)

bismuth subsalicylate (Kaopectate, Pepto-Bismol)

sucralfate (Carafate)

Other

clarithromycin (Biaxin)

metroNIDAZOLE (Flagyl)

misoprostol (Cytotec)

propantheline (Pro-Banthine)

sodium bicarbonate (Baking Soda, Neut)

Proton pump inhibitors (PPIs)

dexlansoprazole (Dexilant)

esomeprazole (NexIUM)

lansoprazole (Prevacid)

omeprazole (PriLOSEC)

pantoprazole (Protonix)

RABEprazole (Aciphex)

Quick Med Fact:

Most PPI's end in "prazole".

Antivirals

DESCRIPTION

These medications are designed to work in one of two ways - they either inhibit the ability to multiply or they mimic the virus attachment protein, disrupting the replication process.

Used to treat:

Prevent, manage and/or treat viral infections, such as HIV, herpes simplex and cytomegalovirus, pneumonia, measles and mumps, and influenza strains (including swine flu).

EXAMPLES

cidofovir (Vistide)

foscarnet (Foscavir)

ganciclovir (Cytovene)

valGANciclovir (Valcyte)

Anti-herpetic agents

acyclovir (Zovirax)

famciclovir (Famvir)

valACYclovir (Valcyte)

Anti-influenza agents

amantadine (Symmetrel)

oseltamivir (Tamiflu)

rimantadine (Flumadine)

zanamivir (Relenza)

Nucleoside analogues

adefovir (Hepsera)

entecavir (Baraclude)

lamiVUDine (Epivir)

penciclovir (Denavir)

ribavirin (Copegus, Rebetol, Virazole)

telbivudine (Tyzeka)

Purine nucleosides

vidarabine (Vira-A)

Quick Med Fact:

Antivirals work best when started within 2 days after becoming ill.

Benzodiazepines

DESCRIPTION

These medications depress the CNS, probably by potentiating GABA, which is an inhibitory neurotransmitter. These are all Schedule IV drugs.

Used to treat:

Produce sedation or induce sleep.

Relieve anxiety and muscle spasms.

Prevent seizures.

EXAMPLES

ALPRAZolam (Xanax)

chlordiazePOXIDE (Librium)

clonazePAM (KlonoPIN)

clorazepate (Tranxene)

diazepam (Valium)

estazolam (ProSom)

flumazenil (Romazicon)

flurazepam (Dalmane)

LORazepam (Ativan)

midazolam (Versed)

oxazepam (Serax)

quazepam (Doral)

temazepam (Restoril)

triazolam (Halcion)

Quick Med Fact:

Long acting benzodiazepines should not be given to the elderly.

Beta-Adrenergic Blocking Agents (Beta Blockers)

DESCRIPTION

These medications block norepinephrine and epinephrine from binding to beta receptors on nerves. By blocking the effects of these neurotransmitters, they reduce heart rate and reduce blood pressure by dilating blood vessels.

Used to treat:

Treat hypertension, heart failure, arrhythmias, and angina (but not for immediate relief).

Treat glaucoma (ophthalmic).

Prevent future heart attacks in heart attack patients.

Prevent migraine headaches.

EXAMPLES

acebutolol (Sectral)

atenolol (Tenormin)

betaxolol (Kerlone)

bisoprolol (Zebeta)

carteolol (Cartrol)

carvedilol (Coreg)

esmolol (Brevibloc)

labetalol (Trandate)

metoprolol (Lopressor, Toprol-XL)

nadolol (Corgard)

nebivolol (Bystolic)

penbutolol (Levatol)

pindolol (Visken)

propranolol (Inderal)

sotalol (Betapace)

timolol (Timoptic

Quick Med Fact:

Usually ends in "LOL"

Bone Resorption Inhibitors

DESCRIPTION

These medications bind to hydroxyapatite in bone and inhibit bone resorption by decreasing the number and activity of osteoclasts.

Used to treat:

Prevent and treat osteoporosis in postmenopausal women and due to other causes, such as Paget's disease of the bone and corticosteroid therapy.

EXAMPLES

alendronate (Fosamax)

calcitonin-salmon (Miacalcin)

etidronate disodium (Didronel)

ibandronate (Boniva)

raloxifene (Evista)

risedronate (Actonel)

tiludronate (Skelid)

Quick Med Fact:

Should be taken on an empty stomach.

Bronchodilators

DESCRIPTION

Medications relax bronchial smooth muscle, enlarging airways and allowing air to pass through the lungs. They may also increase mucociliary clearance (beta agonists).

Used to treat:

Short-acting medications act as asthma "rescue" medications.

Long-acting medications are used to control asthma daily in conjunction with an inhaled steroid.

EXAMPLES

EPINEPHrine (EpiPen, Primatene, Nephron, Adrenalin)

Anticholinergics

ipratropium (Atrovent)

tiotropium (Spiriva)

Beta agonists (long-acting)

arformoterol (Brovana)

formoterol (Foradil)

salmeterol (Serevent)

Beta agonists (short-acting)

albuterol (Proventil, Ventolin, Proair, Accuneb)

levalbuterol (Xopenex)

metaproterenol (Alupent)

pirbuterol (Maxair)

terbutaline (Brethine)

Combination (inhaled steroid + long acting beta agonist)

budesonide & formoterol (Symbicort)

fluticasone & salmeterol* (Advair)

Leukotriene synthesis inhibitors

montelukast* (Singulair)

zafirlukast (Accolate)

zileuton (Zyflo)

Methylxanthines

aminophylline (Phyllocontin, Truphylline)

theophylline (Theo-Dur, Slo-Bid, Aerolate, and others)

Quick Med Fact:

If patient has both inhaled steroid and inhaled bronchodilator, the bronchodilator should be used first.

Calcium Channel Blockers (CCBs)

DESCRIPTION

These medications slow the rate at which calcium passes into the heart muscle and into the vessel walls. This relaxes the vessels and allows blood to flow more easily through them, lowering blood pressure.

Used to treat:

Hypertension, angina, and abnormal heart rhythms (atrial fibrillation, paroxysmal supraventricular tachycardia).

Treat post-MI clients who cannot tolerate beta-blockers.

EXAMPLES

amLODIpine (Norvasc, Lotrel)

bepridil (Vascor)

diltiazem (Cardizem, Dilacor, Tiazac, and others)

felodipine (Plendil)

isradipine (DynaCirc)

niCARdipine (Cardene)

NIFEdipine (Adalat, Procardia XL)

niMODipine (Nimotop)

nisoldipine (Sular)

verapamil (Calan, Covera, Isoptin, Verelan)

Quick Med Fact:

Patients should not eat grapefruit or drink grapefruit juice, this can cause the drug to become toxic.

Central Nervous System Stimulants

DESCRIPTION

Increases physical activity, mental alertness and attention span. The exact mechanism of action is not known.

Used to treat:

Improve concentration and focus for those with attention-deficit hyperactivity disorder (ADHD).

Decrease appetite and promote weight loss.

Alleviate sleep disorders, including narcolepsy, Shift Work Sleep Disorder, and jet lag.

EXAMPLES

amphetamine & dextroamphetamine (Adderall)

benzphetamine (Didrex)

caffeine (NoDoz, Vivarin)

dexmethylphenidate (Focalin)

dextroamphetamine (Dexedrine)

diethylpropion (Tenuate)

lisdexamfetamine (Vyvanse)

methylphenidate (Concerta, Ritalin)

Quick Med Fact:

Can be habit forming.

Can cause sudden death in patients with cardia disorders.

Corticosteroids

DESCRIPTION

Mimics the effect of hormones produced naturally by the adrenal glands. When the dose exceeds the body's usual hormone levels, they will suppress inflammation, as well as the immune system. Also used for their antineoplastic activity.

Used to treat:

Oral forms treat inflammation and pain associated with arthritis and autoimmune diseases (such as lupus, Crohn's).

Inhaled medications treat asthma and allergies.

Topical application helps heal skin conditions.

Injected forms treat the pain and inflammation of arthritis, gout and other inflammatory diseases.

EXAMPLES

beclomethasone (Qvar)

betamethasone (Celestone)

budesonide (Entocort EC, Pulmicort)

cortisone (Cortone Acetate)

dexamethasone (Decadron)

flunisolide (AeroBid)

fluticasone* (Flonase, Flovent)

methylPREDNISolone (Medrol, Depo-Medrol)

mometasone furoate (Nasonex)

prednisoLONE (Orapred, Prelone)

predniSONE (Sterapred)

Quick Med Fact:

Avoid grapefruit and grapefruit juice as it can increase serum levels of thee medications.

Patients taking corticosteroids should not receive live vaccines. They need to contact their healthcare provider first.

Diuretics – Loop

DESCRIPTION

These medications work in the ascending limb of the loop of Henle (where magnesium & calcium are reabsorbed). Disrupted reabsorption causes increased urine production, which lowers blood volume and results in lowered blood pressure. Also causes the veins to dilate, which lowers blood pressure mechanically.

Used to treat:

Acute pulmonary edema and manage edema.

Reduce intracranial pressure and treat hyperkalemia.

EXAMPLES

bumetanide (Bumex)

ethacrynic acid (Edecrin)

furosemide* (Lasix)

torsemide (Demadex)

Quick Med Fact:

Common side effect – hypotension

Patients may require supplemental potassium, folic acid and vitamin B.

Diuretics – Thiazide

DESCRIPTION

These medications are derived from a chemical called benzothiadiazine. They work in the distal convoluted tubule by decreasing the kidney's reabsorption of sodium and chloride (which results in increased urine production) and help dilate blood vessels.

Used to treat:

Hypertension

Edema due to heart failure or other causes.

EXAMPLES

chlorothiazide (Hygroton, Diuril)

hydrochlorothiazide* (HydroDIURIL)

indapamide (Lozol)

metolazone (Zaroxolyn)

Quick Med Fact:

May raise blood sugar levels

Most diuretics drugs contain sulfa – check for allergies prior to giving this medication.

Diuretics – Osmotic

DESCRIPTION

These medications are low-molecular-weight substances that produce a rapid loss of sodium and water by inhibiting their reabsorption in the kidney tubules and the loop of Henle. They increase plasma osmolality, which increases diffusion of water from the intraocular and cerebrospinal fluids.

Used to treat:

Cerebral edema to decrease intracranial pressure.

EXAMPLES

mannitol (Osmitrol)

urea (generic)

Quick Med Fact:

Following administration ICP calls within 60-90 minutes.

Leakage (extravasation) of mannitol can cause necrosis and edema.

Watch for electrolyte imbalances (hypernatremia) from fluid loss.

Diuretics – Potassium-Sparing

DESCRIPTION

Conserves potassium in clients receiving thiazide or loop diuretics. They decrease sodium reabsorption in the collecting tubules of the kidneys.

Used to treat:

Heart failure, as they do not significantly lower blood pressure.

EXAMPLES

aMILoride (Midamor)

eplerenone (Inspra)

spironolactone (Aldactone)

triamterene (Dyrenium)

Quick Med Fact:

NSAIDS can decrease flow of blood to the kidneys and may also interfere with water and sodium excretion, therefore decreasing the effectiveness of the drug.

K+ sparing diuretics have weak diuretic and antihypertensive properties.

Immunizing Agents

DESCRIPTION

Immunizing biological antimicrobial agents (biologicals) are any substance or organism that provokes an immune response when introduced into the body.

Used to prevent:

Infectious diseases.

EXAMPLES

Active immunizing agents

bacille Calmette-Guerin (BCG) vaccine (Theracys)

diphtheria and tetanus toxoids and acellular pertussis adsorbed (DTaP) (Daptacel)

haemophilus b conjugate vaccine (Hib) (ActHIB)

hepatitis A virus vaccine (Havrix, Vaqta)

hepatitis B virus vaccine (Engerix-B)

herpes zoster vaccine* (Zostavax)

human papillomavirus vaccine* (Gardasil)

influenza virus vaccines (many different ones)

measles, rubella, mumps virus vaccine (M-M-R II)

meningococcal polysaccharide bacterial vaccine (Menactra)

poliovirus vaccines (Ipol)

rabies virus vaccine (Imovax Rabies)

rotavirus vaccine (Rotarix)

smallpox virus vaccine (Dryvax)

tetanus toxoid (TE Anatoxal Berna)

typhoid bacterial vaccine (Vivotif)

varicella virus vaccine (Varivax)

yellow fever virus vaccine (YF-VAX)

Passive immunizing agents

antivenin (many different ones)

cytomegalovirus immune globulin (Cytogam)

digoxin immune FAB (DigiFab)

hepatitis B immune globulin (BeyHep B)

rabies immune globulin (BayRab)

respiratory syncytial virus immune globulin (Respigam)

Rho(D) immune globulin (RhoGAM)

tetanus immune globulin (HyperTET S/D)

varicella zoster immune globulin (Varizig)

Quick Med Fact:

Rubella infection can cause miscarriage, stillbirth, birth defects and preterm birth.

Immunosuppressants

DESCRIPTION

Inhibits cell-mediated immune responses.

Used to treat:

Prevent transplantation rejection reactions

Manage selected autoimmune diseases (for example, nephritic syndrome of childhood and severe rheumatoid arthritis).

EXAMPLES

azathioprine (Imuran, Azasan)

basiliximab (Simulect)

chlorambucil (Leukeran)

cyclophosphamide (Cytoxan, Endoxan, Neosar)

cycloSPORINE (Neoral, SandIMMUNE)

daclizumab (Zenapax)

methotrexate (Rheumatrex, Trexall)

muromonab-CD3 (Orthoclone OKT3)

mycophenolate mofetil (CellCept)

mycophenolic acid (Myfortic)

pimecrolimus (Elidel)

sirolimus (Rapamune)

tacrolimus (Prograf)

thalidomide (Thalomid)

Quick Med Fact:

Since these medications lower the body's resistance, patients should not have immunizations. Please check with physician first.

Laxatives

DESCRIPTION

Typically classified as either bulk-forming agents, osmotics, salines, stimulant laxatives or stool softeners.

Used to treat:

Treat or prevent constipation.

Prepare the bowel for radiologic or endoscopic procedures.

EXAMPLES

methylnaltrexone bromide (Relistor)

Bulk-forming agents

polycarbophil (Equalactin, FiberCon)

psyllium (Metamucil)

Osmotics

glycerin suppositories (generic)

lactulose (Chronulac, Cephulac, Cholac)

polyethylene glycol (Miralax)

Salines

magnesium chloride (Mag 64, Mag-SR)

magnesium gluconate (Mag-G, Magonate)

magnesium hydroxide (Milk of Magnesia)

phosphate/biphosphate (Fleet Enema, OsmoPrep)

Stimulant laxatives

bisacodyl (Dulcolax)

sennosides (Senokot)

Stimulant laxatives (Herbal)

aloe (herbal)

Stool softeners

docusate sodium (Colace, Surfak)

Quick Med Fact:

Docusate is usually used after post op procedure or MI to prevent straining while having a bowel movment.

Lipid-Lowering Agents

DESCRIPTION

Reduce LDL "bad" cholesterol by inhibiting the enzyme in the liver (HMG-CoA reductase) responsible for making cholesterol; shrink, stabilize and prevent rupture of fatty plaques and formation of clots; and prevent inflammation (statins).

Reduce LDL by binding to bile acid and preventing absorption of cholesterol from the small intestine (bile acid sequestrants).

Prevent cardiovascular disease in patients with elevated triglycerides and low HDL when diet and lifestyle changes are unsuccessful (fibric acid agents).

Used to treat:

Reduce blood lipids in an effort to reduce the morbidity and mortality of atherosclerotic cardiovascular disease (along with diet and exercise).

EXAMPLES

Bile Acid Sequestrants

cholestyramine (Questran)

colesevelam (Welchol)

colestipol (Colestid)

Fibric Acids

fenofibrate (Tricor)

fenofibric acid (Trilipix)

Gemfibrozil (Lopid)

HMG CoA Reductase Inhibitors

atorvastatin (Lipitor)

pitavastatin (Livalo)

pravastatin (Pravachol)

rosuvastatin (Crestor)

simvastatin (Zocor)

Other

ezetimibe (Zetia)

ezetimibe & simvastatin (Vytorin)

Quick Med Fact:

These are known at "Statins"

Minerals/Electrolytes/pH Modifiers

DESCRIPTION

Correct imbalances minerals and electrolytes or make the urine more alkaline (pH modifiers).

Used to prevent:

Treat or prevent deficiencies or excesses of electrolytes.

Prevent crystals from forming in the urine and inhibit the formation of kidney stones (acidifiers and alkalinizers).

Treat pre-eclampsia and eclampsia (magnesium sulfate).

Some of these meds neutralize gastric acid.

<u>Alkalinizing agents</u>

sodium bicarbonate (Baking Soda, Neut)

<u>Calcium salts</u>

calcium acetate (Eliphos)

calcium carbonate (Caltrate)

 calcium chloride (generic)

calcium citrate (Citracal)

 calcium gluconate (generic)

calcium lactate (Ridactate)

<u>Magnesium salts</u>

magnesium sulfate (generic)

<u>pH modifiers</u>

potassium citrate (Urocit-K)

potassium phosphate (Neutra-Phos-K)

Phosphate supplements

sodium phosphate (OsmoPrep)

Potassium salts

potassium bicarbonate (Effervescent Potassium)

potassium bicarbonate & potassium citrate (K-Lyte)

potassium chloride* (K-Dur, Klor-Con)

Quick Med Fact:

Calcium gluconate is also used as an antidote for magnesium sulfate overdose.

Non-Steroidal Anti-Inflammatory Drugs (NSAIDs)

DESCRIPTION

Blocks the cyclooxygenase (COX-1 & COX-2) enzymes and reduce prostaglandins throughout the body, reducing inflammation, pain, and fever.

Used to treat:

Mild-to-moderate pain, reduce fever, and to treat various inflammatory conditions, such as osteoarthritis.

EXAMPLES

<u>**COX-2 selective inhibitors**</u>

celecoxib (CeleBREX)

<u>**Salicylates**</u>

aspirin (Bayer)

<u>**Traditional NSAIDs**</u>

diclofenac (Cataflam, Voltaren)

diflunisal (Dolobid)

etodolac (Lodine)

ibuprofen (Motrin, Advil)

indomethacin (Indocin)

ketoprofen (Actron, Orudis)

ketorolac (Toradol)

nabumetone (Relafen)

naproxen (Aleve, Naprosyn)

piroxicam (Feldene)

Quick Med Fact:

NSAIDS reduce the ability of the blood to clot.

Ok to take with antacids.

Nonopioid Analgesics

DESCRIPTION

Targets and blocks the chemical substances released by the brain (particularly prostaglandin) in response to injury.

Used to treat:

Mild-to-moderate pain and/or fever.

EXAMPLES

acetaminophen (Tylenol)

chondroitin sulfate (Chondroitin)

phenazopyridine (Pyridium, Urogesic)

salsalate (Amigesic, Disalcid)

Barbiturate + NSAID

butalbital & acetaminophen (Phrenilin)

Botanical medical food

flavocoxid (Limbrel)

Herbals

capsaicin (Icy Hot Arthritis Therapy, ArthriCare for Women)

NSAIDs

choline & magnesium salicylates (Trilisate)

diclofenac (Cataflam, Voltaren)

diflunisal (Dolobid)

etodolac (Lodine)

fenoprofen (Naprofen)

ibuprofen (Motrin, Advil)

ketoprofen (Actron, Orudis)

ketorolac (Toradol)

magnesium salicylate (Doans Pills, Bayer Select Backache Pain Formula)

meclofenamate (Meclomen)

meloxicam* (Mobic)

naproxen* (Aleve, Midol Extended Relief)

Radiopharmaceutical

samarium sm 153 lexidronam (Quadramet)

strontium-89 chloride (Metastron)

Salicylates

aspirin (Bayer)

Quick Med Fact:

Acetaminophen is found in over 500 over the counter drugs.

Opioid Analgesics

These medications interact with opioid receptors in the central nervous system, acting as agonists of endogenously occurring opioid peptides (enkephalins and endorphins). This action alters perception and response to pain. They can be categorized as long-acting, short-acting, or rapid-onset agents.

They are all Schedule II drugs.

Used to treat:

Moderate-to-severe pain.

EXAMPLES

alfentanil (Alfenta)

buprenorphine (Buprenex)

butorphanol (Stadol)

codeine (generic)

fentaNYL (Duragesic)

HYDROcodone (Norco, Vicodin)

HYDROmorphone (Dilaudid, Exalgo)

levorphanol (LevoDromoran)

meperidine (Demerol)

methadone (Dolophine)

morphine (generic)

nalbuphine (Nubain)

oxyCODONE* (OxyContin, Percocet)

oxymorphone (Opana ER)

pentazocine (Talwin)

remifentanil (Ultiva)

SUFentanil (Sufenta)

tapentadol (Nucynta)

traMADol* (Rybix, Ryzolt, Ultram)

Quick Med Fact:

Narcan is a opioid antagonist and should be used in an overdose.

Sedatives/Hypnotics

DESCRIPTION

These medications moderate activity and excitement while inducing a calming effect (and may be anxiolytic). They induce drowsiness and sleep.

Most are Schedule IV drugs.

Used to treat:

Provide sedation, usually prior to procedures.

Selected agents are useful as anticonvulsants, skeletal muscle relaxants, adjuncts in general surgery and adjuncts for the treatment of alcohol withdrawal syndrome.

EXAMPLES

Barbiturates

amobarbital (Amytal)

PENTobarbital (Nembutal)

PHENobarbital (Luminal, Solfoton)

secobarbital (Seconal)

Benzodiazepines (intermediate-acting)

estazolam (ProSom)

LORazepam (Ativan)

temazepam (Restoril)

Benzodiazepines (long-acting)

clorazepate (Tranxene)

diazepam (Valium)

flurazepam (Dalmane)

Benzodiazepines (short-acting)

midazolam (Versed)

oxazepam (Serax)

triazolam (Halcion)

Herbals

chamomile (herbal)

dill (herbal)

kava-kava (herbal)

lemon verbena (herbal)

valerian (herbal)

Other

chloral hydrate (Somnote)

chlordiazePOXIDE (Librium)

dexmedetomidine (Precedex)

droperidol (Inapsine)

eszopiclone (Lunesta)

hydrOXYzine (Atarax, Vistaril)

promethazine (Phenergan)

ramelteon (Rozerem)

zaleplon (Sonata)

zolpidem (Ambien)

Quick Med Fact:

IMPORTANT: even a slight OD of one of the older barbiturates can induce coma and death because of profound CNS depression. But, an overdose of a benzodiazepine or the new non-benzodiazepine sedative hypnotics can typically produce more of an anesthesia effect without risk. Unless combined with alcohol.

Skeletal Muscle Relaxants

DESCRIPTION

Act centrally on the spinal cord or brain stem and inhibit neuronal transmission; dantrolene is the only one that acts directly on skeletal muscle. They are typically classified by their pharmacologic properties as either anti-spasticity or antispasmodic agents.

Used to treat:

Spasticity associated with spinal cord diseases (such as cerebral palsy, multiple sclerosis) or lesions.

Relieve symptoms of acute painful musculoskeletal conditions (as adjunctive therapy).

EXAMPLES

Antispasticity agents

baclofen (Lioresal)

dantrolene (Dantrium)

tiZANidine (Zanaflex)

Musculoskeletal agents

carisoprodol (Soma, Soprodal, Vanadom)

chlorzoxazone (Parafon Forte DSC)

cyclobenzaprine (Flexeril)

metaxalone (Skelaxin)

methocarbamol (Robaxin)

orphenadrine (Norflex)

Other

diazepam (Valium)

Quick Med Fact:

Methocarbamol can cause urine to turn green-black, this is benign and will go away once medication is stopped.

 Carisoprodol is one of the most abused mood altering substance in the U.S.

Dantrolene is used to treat and prevent malignant hyperthermia.

Thrombolytics

DESCRIPTION

Converts plasminogen to plasmin, which then degrades fibrin in clots.

Used to manage:

Coronary thrombosis (MI), massive pulmonary emboli, deep vein thrombosis, and arterial thromboembolism.

EXAMPLES

alteplase (Activase)

reteplase (Retavase)

streptokinase (Streptase)

tenecteplase (TNKase)

urokinase (Abbokinase)

Quick Med Fact:

Aminocaproic acid may be used as an antidote.

If Alteplase is used to manage acute ischemic stroke in adults, it should be initiated within 3 hours of onset of symptoms, unless other contraindications exist.

Tocolytic Agents

DESCRIPTION

These medications inhibit uterine contractions and suppress pre-term labor.

Used to teat:

Pre-term labor.

EXAMPLES

magnesium sulfate (MgSO4) (generic)

Beta-mimetics

terbutaline (Brethine)

Calcium Channel Blockers

nifedipine (Adalat, Procardia)

Non-Steroidal Anti-Inflammatory Drugs

indomethacin (Indocin)

Quick Med Fact:

Effective in stopping labor for 48-72 hours, this will allow the healthcare team to plan other interventions to improve outcome.

** Terbutaline carries a black box warning regarding its use as a tocolytic. Prolonged use over 48 hours can be associated with hyperglycemia, cardiac problems, hypokalemia, and death.

Vascular Headache Suppressants

DESCRIPTION

Stimulates alpha-adrenergic and serotonergic receptors, producing vascular smooth muscle vasoconstriction (ergot derivatives).

Narrow dilated blood vessels and block nerves from transmitting signals of pain to the brain (5-HT1 agonists).

Used to treat:

Vascular headaches (migraines and cluster headaches).

EXAMPLES

5-HT1 agonists

almotriptan (Axert)

eletriptan (Relpax)

frovatriptan (Frova)

naratriptan (Amerge)

rizatriptan (Maxalt)

SUMAtriptan (Imitrex)

ZOLMitriptan (Zomig)

Beta blockers

propranolol (Inderal)

timolol (Timoptic)

Calcium channel blocker

verapamil (Calan, Covera, Isoptin, Verelan)

Ergots

dihydroergotamine (D.H.E. 45)

ergotamine (Ergomar)

Herbals

feverfew (herbal)

Quick Med Fact:

Seritonin receptor agonists "triptans" do not prevent migraines. They will prevent symptoms from getting worse.

Vasopressors

DESCRIPTION

Potent vasoconstrictors that produce a rise in blood pressure (specifically, an increase in mean arterial pressure).

Used to treat:

Hypotensive states, such as (cardiogenic, septic) shock, drug reactions, spinal anesthesia.

Prolong anesthesia.

Treat certain heart rhythm problems, including cardiac arrest.

EXAMPLES

DOPamine (generic)

EPINEPHrine (EpiPen, Primatene, Nephron, Adrenalin)

midodrine (ProAmatine)

norepinephrine (Levophed)

phenylephrine (Neo-Synephrine)

Quick Med Fact:

Administer in large veins such as the antecubital vein.

Vitamins

DESCRIPTION

These organic compounds, present in minute amounts in foods, are essential for normal growth and development. Fat-soluble vitamins are stored in the liver and excreted via the feces; water-soluble vitamins are not stored in the body and are excreted in the urine.

Uses:

Dietary supplement.

Treat vitamin deficiency.

Treat skin conditions.

EXAMPLES

Fat soluble

cholecalciferol/D3 (Drisdol, Calciferol)

vitamin A (Lumitene, Aquasol A, Retinol)

vitamin E (Aquasol E, Aquavite-E)

vitamin K (Mephyton, AquaMephyton)

Water soluble

ascorbic acid/C (Cenolate, Vita C)

B-complex vitamin (Slo-Niacin)

cyanocobalamin/B12 (CaloMist, Nascobal)

folic acid (Folvite)

niacin/B3 (Niacor, Niaspan)

pyridoxine/B6 (Aminoxin, Nestrex)

thiamine/B1 (Thiamilate)

Nursing Pharmacology Exam with Rationale

To complete the computer based 100 question exam, please go to:

http://nursestudy.net/pharmacology-100-test/

Disclaimer

Nursing and medicine are continuously changing and evolving. All the information in this publication have been reviewed for accuracy. The information in this publication are believed to be reliable and accurate. However, despite all efforts and continual changes in best practices, the publisher and author, and any other party involved in the production of this information disclaim all responsibility from any mistakes and errors contained within the work and from the results of the use of this information. Readers are encouraged to check all information and institutional policies for up to date guidelines.

This book is not intended to provide medical advice. The articles in this publication are intended for educational value only. While we strive to offer 100% accuracy, we cannot guarantee the validity or accuracy of any content. Medical procedures are rapidly changing, and laws vary greatly from location to location. We also allow user-submitted content on this site, such as personal medical experiences or opinions, or tips on nursing school or nursing procedures. By viewing or accessing this book in any way, you agree to never us liable for any damages, harm, or misinformation that may result, and that you fully agree with our legal disclosure and privacy policy. Copyright Notice: All articles, eBooks, images, and information on this website is copyright protected and property of our website. You may not copy any information without our expressed written consent.

NCLEX®, NCLEX®-RN®, and NCLEX®-PN® are registered trademarks of the National Council of State Boards of Nursing, Inc. They hold no affiliation with this book or related products.